Essential Oils:

25 Essential Oils Recipes for Kids

Table of Contents

Introduction: Just Follow Your Nose

The concept of utilizing fragrant oils to treat disease has been with us for thousands of years. With essential oils having a history that dates back for over five thousand. It was in India that such practices were finely perfected into the healing practice of Ayurvedic medicine. In ancient India all you had to do was follow your nose and you could be led to healing essential oil.

But this precious oil didn't remain unique to just India, because since then oils of all kind of been extracted from roots, leaves, fruits, and even flowers, and have been used for all kinds of benefit and purpose all over the world. We are approaching the Christmas season now, and every child knows the story of the three wise men that brought Frankincense and Myrrh to the baby Jesus. They would also be interested to know that Frankincense and Myrrh are two of the most famous and powerful essential oils ever put under a Christmas tree!

Even before that first Christmas story, Frankincense and Myrrh was a sacred sacrament of the temple in Israel in which the strong aroma was used as incense to bring the children of Israel into the right state mind of mind and bring about mental focus. These essential oils and many others like them can still be used to bring about that central clarity and focus in our children today. Known to treat everything from ADHD to anxiety and depression, in order to find a solution for many of the problems that our kids face today, all you really have to do is just follow your nose!

Chapter 1: Use of Essential Oil For Health and Relaxation

The most important thing to learn about Essential Oils is how to apply. You need to be careful—especially when it comes with your kids—not to use too much. In this chapter we are going to explore all of the various methods that can be used in which to apply the healing power of essential oil. There are several benefits that can be derived from essential oils and here are a few.

Using Carrier Oil

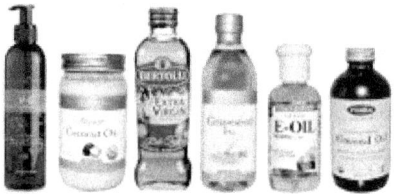

Essential oils are typically pretty highly concentrated, and just a few drops are usually enough to mete out their benefit. And since just a few drops is all you will need, you will have to learn how to apply it through a diluted compound known as a "carrier oil". With just a few drops mixed in with other base oils such as "Olive Oil", or even "Baby Oil" you can then just massage the combined mixture into the skin to alleviate whatever affliction your kids are suffering from.

This method is a great way to help kids with hyperactivity and relaxation issues. With this kind of treatment you can stimulate the lymph nodes, increasing the flow of blood and oxygen, directly to the brain. This application method also has a direct link to removing toxins from the body and even lowering the pressure of the blood. What's even better is that this method has been shown to increase mental focus in those who use it.

Applying Essential Oil Through Diffusion

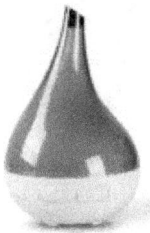

Along with the use of carrier oils, another great way to bring benefit from essential oils is to use an application method known as "diffusion". This method employs another variation of aromatherapy, in order to spread the fragrance of an essential oil around the room by diffusing its potency over a wide range of space. This is a great method for kids who have trouble sleeping for example, and you wish to spread a fragrant oil that helps put them to sleep.

But diffusion can serve many purposes, such as helping t alleviate stress, chronic coughing, and even as a disinfectant. The most popular way to diffuse essential oil is by burning them as incense. A properly diffusing method of essential oil dispersal has even been used as a kind of nebulizer for asthma sufferers. Another method of application for essential oil that is very similar to that of diffusion, is simply to directly inhale the oil right into the nose.

For direct inhalation, no heating is needed and administration can be as simple as just taking the cap off of the bottle of essential oil and having your child inhale the aroma. Alternatively you could also place a drop of essential oil in their bath-water so that they can breathe it in while they take a bath. Just keep in mind that since these essential oils are fairly powerful in their concentration, always make sure their use is supervised. Only allow them to do this when you are around to administer it, and always keep your essential oils in a safe place.

Using an Aromatic Compress

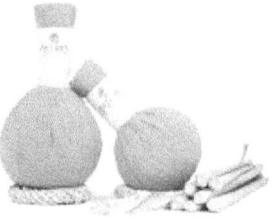

And finally, one more good method of essential oil application is that of the "aromatic compress". You can use this method to place essential oil in cold icepack-like compresses, aimed at alleviating a wide range of aches, fever, bruises and burns. With an aromatic compress you can put as much healing power as you can within one tightly condensed area. This provides a very potent and immediate treatment. These are all great methods for the application of essential oils!

Chapter 2: Best Essential Oils for Health and Wellness

In this chapter let's now dive right into that list of the 25 most essential oils that you can use. There are quite a few great blends that can be used for many different purposes for health and wellness, especially when it comes to anxiety and depression. The categories that these 25 oils come from can be broken down into 8 main groups; earthy, woody, spicy, resinous, camphoraceous, herbaceous, floral, and citrus. Let's explore these further.

Rose Oil

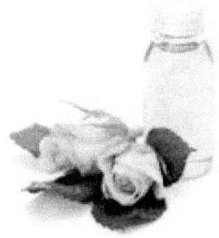

Hailing from the floral family, rose makes for a beautiful flower, and once its oil is extracted it can also make for an enriching and healing essential oil. Rose oil is good at calming and relaxing anxious feelings. If your child is especially hyper, rose oil may be of use. Rose is also works as an immune booster and an anti-viral agent, so it is definitely worth administering as a multipurpose health aid. In order to create your own rose oil, simply take 2 drops of this essential oil and mix it with vegetable or baby oil, and then apply directly to the skin. After a few moments whatever pent up angst that your kids are feeling will surely disappear. So when they are feeling extra hyped up, just let them have some rose oil!

Geranium Oil

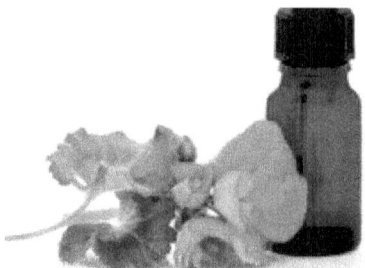

This essential oil works well as an antiviral agent, alleviating any viruses your kids get. It is especially helpful during the cold and flu season. If your kids are feeling a bit under the weather, just have them inhale a bit of Geranium oil and it will give them just the boost they need. Geranium oil has also been known to help with depression and insomnia. So if your children are having a particularly rough not, just administer some Geranium oil right before they go to sleep.

This oil is based used with diffusion. Just add a few drops t an incense burner in or just outside your child's room and they can benefit from the aroma. If they are feeling a little bit down after school just have this geranium oil burning and as soon as they come in the door their spirits will be lifted. This oil can leave a re-membered psychological imprint and become a great way to elevate moods even on bad days.

Due to this mood elevating ability, this essential oil has been found to actually help those that suffer from "seasonal affective disorder" (SAD), the disorder in which people are affected by loss of sunlight and the change of the seasons from warm summer to cold winter. So when they come in all bummed out from the cold keep the home fires burning with some geranium oil and you can lift their spirits right up!

Lotus Oil

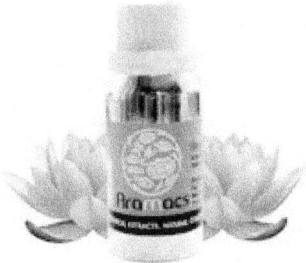

This essential oil is actually great for alleviating the symptoms of childhood asthma. Just a few deep breaths of it's fragrant aroma is enough to pen up the air passages, and get fresh blood flowing, reinvigorating the body. This then also initiates a kind of relaxation response that calms the body and the mind.

Use this essential oil through a recipe of 2 drops placed in carrier oil and then burned as mild incense aroma. If your child is having an asthma attack or just feeling short of breath, you can start treating them with the vapors of this essential oil. If your child's feelings of shortness of breath persist however, be sure to seek medical help immediately. Use this essential oil as needed.

Jasmine Oil

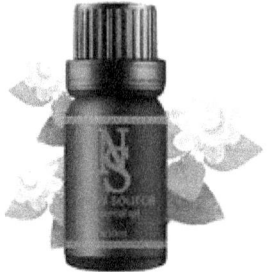

The fragrance of Jasmine essential oil does wonders in alleviating bouts of child-hood anxiety and depression, and other signs of mental exhaustion. One of the secrets of Jasmine's potency stems fro the fact that its oil is extracted rather rapidly from the flower, leaving it in a rather purified condition. Jasmine is best administered by rubbing it directly into the skin.

The recipe for Jasmine essential oil calls for just 2 drops of this oil placed in a carrier solution such as vegetable oil. Then simply have it lightly massaged into the shoulders. The chemical compounds of this oil then go straight to the brain to bring back clarity and relieve fatigue. Kids can sometime be tired immediately before and after school, sometimes a little bit of boost is all they need, essential jasmine oil can revive their senses and give them that extra boost. Jasmine essential oil is a powerful ally to have on your side.

Neroli Oil

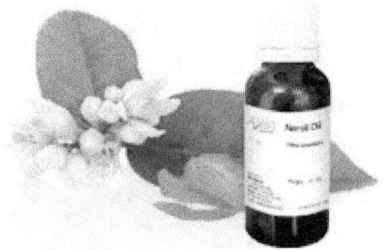

This essential oil has been particularly helpful for parents of children with ADHD. Known as a natural calming agent, neroli can actually decrease rapid heart beats, and calm hyperactive body's and mind's. Place 3 drops of this oil into a carrier base and then gently massage it into the skin in order to see the best results.

I had bouts of ADHD myself as a child and was introduced to this essential oil as an alternative to pharmaceutical treatment. I never really cared for the over the counter medication for ADHD, so once I heard of this alternative I was ready to try it. I wasn't disappointed. If your kids are having trouble paying attention you should give neroli oil a try. You will be amazed at the results you will see.

Marigold Oil

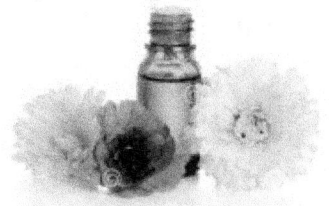

This oil from the Marigold flower can work as a wonderful antiseptic. And if your kids scrape their knees just a few drops of this oil applied with a carrier base to the surface of the sore works well to treat such wounds. Marigold has also been well documented in its use of treating anxiety. Just apply to the skin as much as needed. This essential oil is just as soothing to the skin as it is to the mind and body. Apply liberally and as needed.

Grapefruit Oil

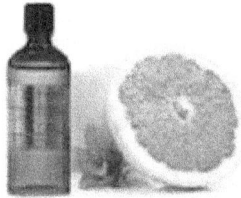

Grapefruits are a healthy treat and the essential oil extracted from it has some amazing properties. This oil is known for its incredible ability to alleviate headaches, cramps, and other aches and pains. If your little one is complaining of a bad headache just have them rub some of this grapefruit oil directly on their forehead and they will be feeling better in no time. The soothing recipe for Grapefruit oil requires 3 drops of this extract mixed with a carrier base. Just apply directly to the skin and you should see some results right away. It doesn't take much effort to make or apply this essential oil, so give it a try!

Tangerine Oil

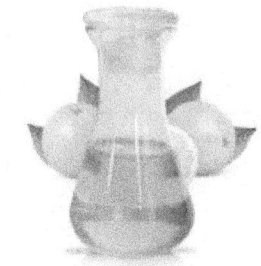

Great for its calming affect, if you've got a young one who is a bit rambunctious just have them rub this tangerine oil into their hands and they will soon begin the process of calming down. It just takes 2 drops of this oil with a carrier base, and you will see some truly fantastic results. The tangerine oil has special compounds that can help to substantially soothe the nerves.

Lime Oil

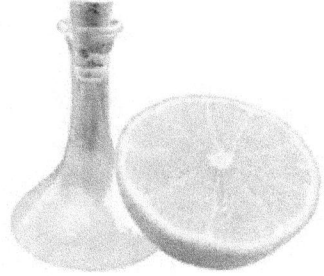

Lime Oil is loaded with Vitamin C and this is good news if your kids have a bad cold. If they are sniffling and sneezing, just put a couple drops of lime oil on a spoon and have them breathe in the fragrance. Lime is refreshing and it is a natural immune booster, this immune boost can shield your kids from the flu and other illnesses that are so prevalent in their schools certain times of year. So be sure to stock up on some lime oil just for that contingency.

Chapter 3: Essential Oil for Stomach and Digestive Health

If your kid's tummy is frequently bothering them, you may want to look into essential oil treatments for what ails them. It's natural, it doesn't have any side effects and it won't break your budget. If your kids are having stomach or other digestive health issues, don't delay; have them put on an essential oil regimen today!

Fennel Oil

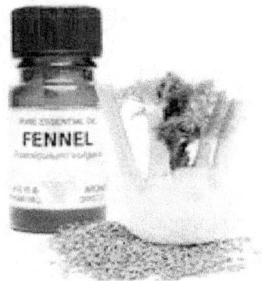

Fennel oil is extracted from fennel seeds through a process o steam distillation. Fennel essential oil has many good uses. Fennel essential oil can work as a mouth freshener as well as a stomach pain reliever. It is for the treatment of stomach pain that you may find the most beneficial aspect of this essential oil, because with just a little bit of this oil, even the most acute stomach cramping can be alleviated.

Fennel oil delivers a strong message to the digestive system. Fennel essential oil has been found to cure even the most persistent of stomach and esophageal ailments. Interestingly, Fennel Oil presents itself even as a cure to the hiccups! If your child is struggling with any of these issues simply have them breathe in a few drops of this oil diffused with incense. If there stomach is making them sick, just a little bit of fennel oil will certainly do the trick!

Rosemary Oil

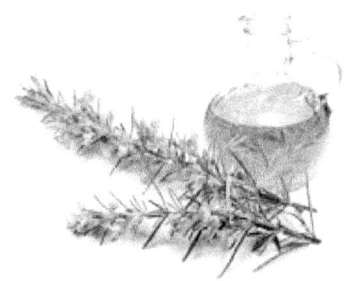

Rosemary is a great asset for stomach health. Rosemary has a knack for stopping many digestive issues in right in its tracks, a quick action response that many digestive sufferers need, especially when it comes to the onset of diarrhea. If your child is suffering from diarrhea just have them inhale the aroma of rosemary oil and it will immediately get to work as an anti-diarrheal agent. Just put 2 drops of rosemary into an incense burner and have your kids inhale the fragrance. This treatment will soon put your kids at ease.

Peppermint Oil

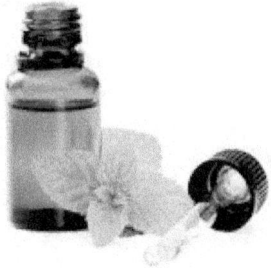

The use of peppermint oil can greatly benefit the gut, freeing the stomach from flatulence, cramps and other digestive problems. If your child is having digestive issues, have them simply breathe in some peppermint and it will instantly help them to relax their stomach, aiding in digestion and using the bathroom. Peppermint is a great nonintrusive treatment, with a pleasant aroma, it's hand down better than many other alternatives.

Lemon Oil

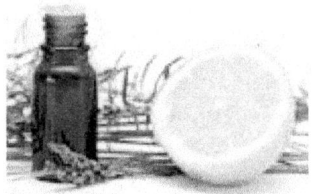

Great for an all around reset of the digestive oil, lemon oil refreshes the hole body. Lemmon oil is also good for the treatment of constipation. If your child is having trouble going to the bathroom, you can have them breathe in a few drops of lemon oil in order to help them go. Take three drops and use an incense diffuser to spread the aroma around the room. Lemon oil will work to break up the malaise of your kids digestive system.

Lavender Oil

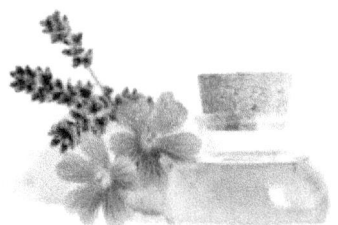

Lavender Oil is a natural muscle relaxer, and it can do wonders for an upset stomach. Just apply 2 drops of lavender oil in a base carrier oil and have your kids rub it into their neck and arms. The lavender oil will then be quickly absorbed and get right to work in relaxing their stomach. This is a soothing blend that can make all the difference in the world when it comes to stomach trouble. Always keep some lavender oil around.

Frankincense Oil

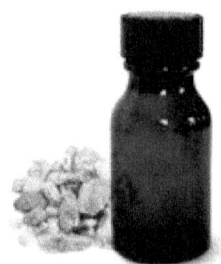

This gift of the Magi; frankincense oil has been around or a long time, and it has been put to great use for centuries. Frankincense works great to reduce inflammation and also works as a way to detox the entire body. If your kid is having stomach trouble just have them rub a couple drops of frankincense oil on their neck and chest and they will be feeling better in no time. Frankincense was good enough for the three wise men, and it can be good enough for your kids! Give this essential oil a try!

Chamomile Oil

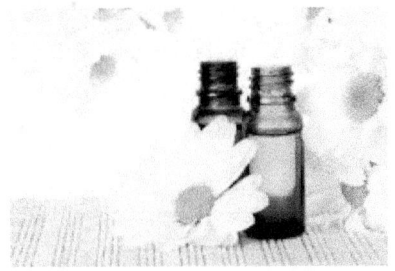

This essential oil can work to greatly relax the smooth muscle fibers of the digestive system. It is also known to be a cure for restlessness and anxiety. So if you have a child whose stomach or body is otherwise unsettled, you can just let them breathe in a few drops of chamomile oil. This essential oil is a great boon to a sluggish digestive system. So in order to jump start your kid's stomachs, you may want to have them give it a try. Chamomile soothes and heals!

Bergamot Oil

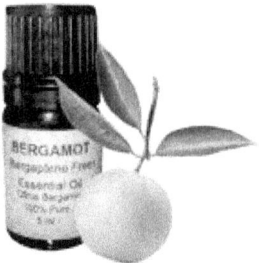

This oil works as an antispasmodic, relieving stomach cramps as well as digestive issues. Bergamot also works to stimulate bile and insulin production greatly aiding digestion. Another great use of bergamot is as an antibacterial agent, since its components kill many harmful bacteria on contact. Having that said, one of the best ways to apply bergamot is to mix it together with dish soap and have your kids wash their hands with it. They will feel better in no time!

Ginger Oil

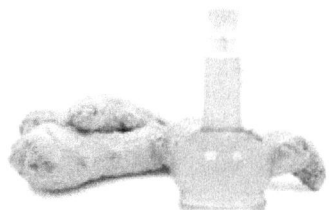

If you do much cooking you may be familiar with ginger. But more than just a cooking ingredient, this herb can produce a powerful essential oil that cures nausea and upset stomach. In order to use ginger oil place 2 drops in a small bowl of hot water. You can microwave your water beforehand in order to make it hot. Have your kids sit at the table right in front of the steaming bowl so they can breathing in the healing vapors of the ginger oil as he steams of the surface o the water. After about five minutes of this their feelings of nausea will be greatly reduced, if not eliminated completely.

Coriander Oil

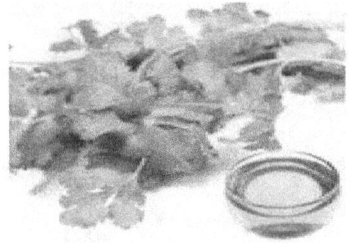

The main benefit of coriander oil is not exactly pleasant but many have trouble with it; gas. Yep, that's right, if your children are particularly gaseous just give them a batch of coriander oil and it will clear that problem up right away! Coriander oil has an amazing way allowing built up gas in the digestive system safe passage—elsewhere!

Just put two drops of this oil in an incense burner, have your kids breathe in the aroma nearby, and hopefully their own gaseous aroma will soon vacate the area! You will also find that coriander is good at regaining overall health and balance to the stomach. These are all good reasons to keep some coriander oil and all the other essential oils presented in this chapter, around for your kids for when they need them.

Chapter 4: Some Special Oil Mixes

In this chapter we would like to introduce you to some special recipe mixes, that take the best of two different oils and combines them together! Check out all of these great blends and put them to great use for you and your kids!

Orange Lavender Oil

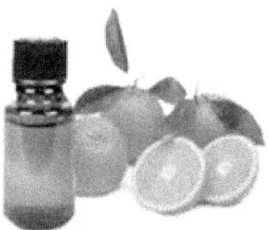

If your kids are having trouble with restlessness and anxiety, you can give them this special essential oil blend t calm them down. To make this one, take 14 drops of clary sage, 9 drops of sweet orange oil, along with 4 drops of lavender oil. Just apply this mixture directly to the skin, and you will feel a cool and relaxing effect that will work its way all throughout the body. The special ingredients of lavender take root in the human body and almost immediately start to take away those jitters. I can remember my own mother giving me this treatment before the first day of school just to take the edge off. It works like a charm!

Ylang Ylang with a Hint of Jasmine Oil

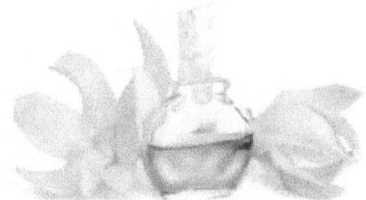

Another soothing blend can be created when you combine 14 drops of ylang ylang, along with 4 drops of jasmine. This concoction does wonders to relieve stress. If your kids have had a particularly bad day, or are just having a bad case of the jitters, let them have this blend of essential oil. Simply apply directly to skin as needed and they will feel a lot better for it.

Roman Chamomile Blended Oil

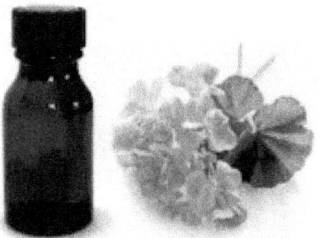

This blend of essential oil works splendidly well for a nighttime aid when your young ones are trying to sleep. Just take 14 drops of Roman Chamomile oil and then blend it with 4 drops of Ylang Ylang for that extra kick. Just have them rub this special oil into their hands and administer as needed. It works great!

Cypress Mix Oil

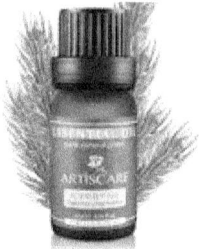

This is a soothing blend consisting of 4 drops of rosemary, 9 drops of lavender, and 14 drops of cypress. This combination works well to alleviate headaches and many minor aches and pains. In order to administer this oil simply steam it and allow them to breathe in the aroma, it will then settle down into their system in no time, working to eliminate those bad aches and pains.

Nutmeg and Neroli Oil

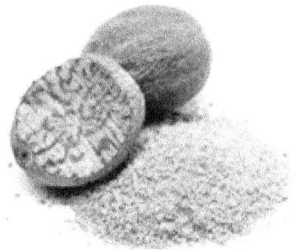

This one requires a pretty special combination of 11 drops of neroli, 15 drops of pettigraine, and 7 drops of nutmeg. When these ingredients are combined, they serve to create a very relaxing blend, for anyone on a stressful day. To administer this combination place the main components in a carrier oil and then distribute into an incense burner to diffuse the material liberally into the room.

Coconut Grape Oil

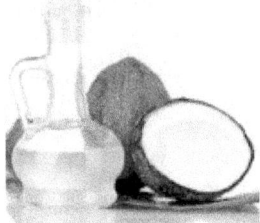

With just a couple drops of coconut and grape oil mixed together you can come up with some great benefits. This blend provides some very specific antimicrobial elements that are great in dealing with harmful stomach bacteria and parasites. The best way to administer this oil is to apply it with a carrier base and then burn it with incense. As soon as you breathe it in, your stomach will thank you for it!

Chapter 5: How to Find the Most Essential of Oils

In this guide we have discussed at great length the ingredients and specific uses f 25 different kinds of essential oils. Now let's answer what may be the most glaring question for many; where do you find essential oils? In the past the options may have been much more limited, but you will find that right here in the present is the best place to be in the search for finding the most essential of oils. In this chapter let's go over some of the best places to find this precious resource.

Online Distributers

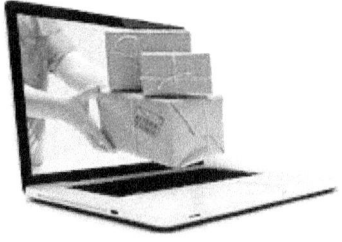

There are in fact, many options to choose from online when it comes to essential oil. In fact with just a few well aimed Google searches you should be able to find many vendors to choose from. Finding a vendor is not a problem, the main challenge that you will face is to make sure that the vendor is in fact selling a quality product. In doing this, there are a few basic pieces of criteria that you should look out for. Most important among these, is the grade of the oil.

Among the most common grade that you might encounter are, perfumed oil, fragrant oil, perfume grade oil and pure grade oil. You need to be able to inundate yourself with the nuances that these classifications imply. If you see something that is "identical grade" for example, this means the essential oil that you are looking at is essentially made to be "identical" to another brand.

In other words, it is generic. But then if you see something listed as "pure grade" this means that it is a highly concentrated form of essential oil and not merely a diluted form that is meant to mimic or be nearly identical to the real thing. Perfume oil is somewhere in the middle when it comes to potency and just like the name describes it is a fragrant water based solution very much akin to other store bought perfumes.

Perfume oil is fairly diluted, but even more watered down than this would be the grade that barely qualifies as essential oil, called, "floral water grade". Floral water grade has such a low potency that it is unable to make much of an effect therapeutically. Floral water grade is usually used simply as a base for other materials, as is the case with most consumer brand makeup and lotions.

When you are buying your essential oils you should pay particular attention to the grade of what you are buying, making sure that it is of a sufficient standard. It may help you to note that, more powerful grade oils are typically housed in nondescript brown bottles, either with eyedropper or standard lids. So keep an eye out for these in particular, especially when you are buying things online, make sure you know the grade before you have the product shipped out!

Buying Off the Counter at Local Stores

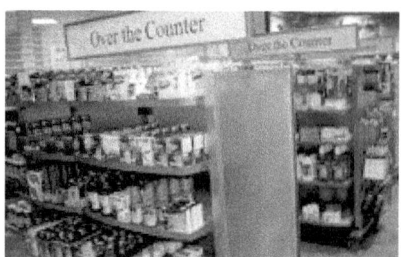

As great as online shopping is, sometimes nothing beats being able to browse your options first hand in a brick and mortar store. And there are a lot of great in person opportunities around when it comes to acquiring essential oils. Some personal favorites of mine include, but are not limited to, "Trader Joes, GMC, Vitamin Shoppe, and Whole Foods.

These places are always fun to shop around in with their laid back, casual atmosphere, and often enough they even provide some oil samples without even having to make a purchase. Just go to a Vitamin Shoppe on the weekend and you are liable to be treated with all kinds of freebies. So it's always worth a visit.

Just remember that price often depends on whether the product is from a retailer or wholesales, a store like Whole Foods might actually have both, with some products being pitched for the little guy as well as big name corporations. Because when you can go for the little guy, because they usually have the best bargains, since they are selling direct. I hope this chapter has helped you in your search for where you can find essential oils!

Conclusion: In Need of an Oil Change!

In the world of today, our kid's face many challenges. Whether in their social life or in their academic life, they are having to learn many new things. But it becomes much harder to learn when they have physical and mental ailment that robs them of their focus and mental clarity. These distractions can wreak havoc on their daily routine.

And the more they progress in this unbalanced state the more unbalanced they get, creating a dangerous cycle that perpetually repeats itself. But you can be the one who puts an end to these risky repetitions and reinstitutes the health and wellness of your child. Your kids can benefit from essential oil treatments, because just like a car needs a tune up after so many miles, your kids just might be in some serious need of an oil change.

FREE Bonus Reminder

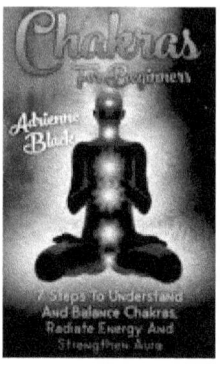

If you have not grabbed it yet, please go ahead and download your special bonus E book *"Chakras for Beginners. 7 Steps To Understand And Balance Chakras, Radiate Energy, And Strengthen Aura"*.

Simply Click the Button Below

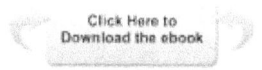

OR Go to This Page

http://lifehacksworld.com/free

BONUS #2: More Free & Discounted Books & Products

Do you want to receive more Free/Discounted Books or Products?

We have a mailing list where we send out our new Books or Products when they go free or with a discount on Amazon. Click on the link below to sign up for Free & Discount Book & Product Promotions.

=> Sign Up for Free & Discount Book & Product Promotions <=

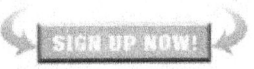

OR Go to this URL